EAT, DRINK, AND GET THIN

Eat, Drink, and Get Thin

ERNST R. REINSH, M.D.

HART PUBLISHING COMPANY, INC.
NEW YORK CITY

To my wife

Contents

EAT, DRINK, AND GET THIN

The Low-Down on Starvation Diets

1

THE ODDS ARE LONG that if you are reading this book you weigh more than you would like to—or ought to. The odds are just about as long that you have experimented again and again with reducing diets foisted upon you by poor misled souls, diets which have actually deprived you of your one best hope of reducing.

The exponents of starvation, the condemners of fatty foods and all else that can give you more than momentary relief from hunger's pangs, have been doing you a disservice. Their promise is that if you starve you will shrivel—which you assuredly will. But as you have already learned through anguished experience, you will stay shriveled only so long as you can steel yourself against those incessant pangs.

Obesity control, as the starvationists conceive it, has to be perpetual martyrdom. Among the hundreds who come to me, this essaying of a martyr's existence is a familiar story. Equally familiar is one's inability to stay with it. Who could? Let obesity's multiple evils be what they may, the starving person persistently finds his plight as a fat man a far better choice than an unending vista of wafers and watercress.

Anyone can lose weight—lots of it. All a man has to do is starve himself. If he lacks willpower to forego nourishment when it is all about him, there are alternatives. For instance, he can arrange to become lost in a desert, or in an abandoned coal mine.

The trouble is that such debilitating rigors most often turn out to have short-lived salutary effects; in fact, such a regimen may be permanently ruinous to one's health. Many of us surely know someone who "has never been the same" after striving to stay alive for a considerable period of time on prisoner-of-war rations.

Voluntary starvation is not medically advisable—at least, not for a protracted length of time. The human system makes no distinction between the consequences of food unavailable and food refused. Were this not so, there would be no need to forcibly feed an individual who goes on a hunger strike.

Of course, if starvation is not too protracted, lasting harm seldom results. In a short time, the victim is himself again— which means, among other things, that he has regained the poundage he carried before his ordeal. The only time the weight does not come back once the starvation process has ceased is after general and permanent damage has been done.

This is precisely why a person who puts himself on a diet which gives less nourishment than he needs will find his former weight returning as soon as he stops adhering to his diet. And precisely why—if he hasn't stopped his foolishment soon enough—he finds himself saddled with indispositions and enfeeblements. For as doctors know and laymen seldom realize, obesity is a disease whose control calls for sound and permanent measures.

Let me emphasize that *random methods of control, such as do-it-yourself calorie counting, sitting in steam cabinets, or lying on massage tables, will produce no lasting benefit.*

Let me interpolate here that in my practice I deal only with people who are seriously overweight. I am not talking about such individuals who carry a few more pounds than they would prefer to during the Bikini season. Nor do I treat them. The weight fluctuation in their cases can be managed by themselves. I am concerned with the many who are authentic obesity sufferers, who put on pounds right and left. I am concerned with the thousands who are now, so to speak, on their 24th semi-annual diet. I am concerned with the myriads who undergo constant torture—either the torture of deprivation, or the torture of guilt and shame.

Starvation diets remind me of the farmer's mule that was gradually being accustomed to getting along without eating at all. It was a great idea but the mule finally betrayed its owner by dying.

The reason you are overweight is that your furnace has not been working at anything like its best efficiency. The fact is that your furnace will hardly work well, if all it gets is low-combustion fuel rationed out by the gram. In such a situation, the body has no choice but to eat itself—that is, as long as the tissues and the organs last. In a starvation regimen, you eat up your own body, and I don't believe that's good for you.

The Insidious Onset

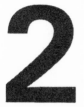

THE GREAT EPIDEMIC of American obesity started about 50 years ago. Generally speaking, we were a Slim Jim nation until somewhat after World War I. Up to then, obesity was so far from being a national characteristic that the problem was of small concern to the medical profession.

At the start of the twentieth century, the overweight person was a rarity, to be encountered mainly among those middle-aged Americans who were physically inactive, and able to dine and drink a good deal more sumptuously than the average citizen. Such a person was called portly, and is envisioned as having worn a heavy gold chain across a dignified expanse of waistcoat.

But the typical individual of that era could not escape activity. While he usually had plenty to eat, it was what was called "good plain food."

People fat in the Falstaffian manner were so uncommon as to be almost freaks, and were certainly memorable. General Shafter, who led our Cuban expeditionary force in 1898, is at least as well recollected for bulk as for generalship. A historian would no more think of omitting reference to Shafter's nearly 300 pounds than he would consider omitting Teddy Roosevelt's performance at San Juan Hill.

There are few today who can tell you anything about William Howard Taft's administration, yet everyone knows that President Taft was fat. Girth such as Taft carried was such a rarity that it endowed him with lasting identity to the public mind.

What has changed all this? What has made obesity an American characteristic so prevalent that how to lose weight has become one of the country's leading preoccupations? Americans have always tended to be a nation of hearty eaters; witness the farmer's loaded table, the heavy breakfasts, the big noonday dinners, banquets with rich courses succeeding each other until midnight, church suppers with three kinds of pie and six kinds of cake. Yet despite a heavy intake, our forbears did not turn out to be over-upholstered men and women. How did they keep their weight down?

Clues why more and more Americans were becoming too heavy for their own good began coming my way very early in my professional career. With these clues plus consistent observation and reading, I learned the medically correct way to bring people back to normal weight and keep them there.

A leading factor in bringing on the obesity epidemic came with the addition of iodine to table salt. Iodine, it was found, could suppress goiter. Fluoride added to water may well have the same effect.

Now don't, for heaven's sake, start shopping for salt that is not iodized. None but the most eccentric food faddist would contest the wisdom of what amounts to a public health measure. Because today we are a people virtually free of goiter, there is scant appreciation nowadays of how prevalent that condition used to be. The discovery that goiter could be done away with simply by putting a bit of iodine in our salt was a truly great victory for the medical profession and for the food industry.

But great as the blessing of iodinizing has been, the benefit of iodine has been realized at the expense of altering our glandular action. While making our glands do one thing, iodine has had the side effect of lowering the thermostat which controls the starch-burning furnace. Suppressed glandular activity through the use of iodine is, I am convinced, the original cause of our nation growing fat.

Just about the time that iodine became a salt additive, the food industry began to ply us with legions of starch-laden goodies. Thus, just when our natural ability to dispose of excess starch was being decreased through the ingestion of iodine, we began to take in vastly increased quantities of starch.

And by far the greater part of the food industry's sales pitch is directed toward tempting us to take into our systems still more obesity-generating starch. Witness the proliferation of ads for spaghetti, cakes, pies, breads, muffins, cookies, crackers, etc. No bets are missed. The Madison Avenue Boys have latched on to bread sliced at the bakery, ready-mixed recipes which promise better cakes than mother used to make, and even macaroni casseroles. This kind of mouth-watering palaver has created a new generation of fatties.

The answer to why so many Americans are overweight lies not nearly so much in the quantity of food they eat, as it does in the kinds of food they now eat.

How I Came
to the High-Fat Diet

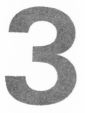

I WAS BROUGHT UP on a Nebraska farm. Hard physical exertion brought me to the family table with a hearty appetite. I ate on the scale of a robust adult. And what I ate principally was home-slaughtered pork—fat and rich. It was what we had the most of.

According to the countless variants of reducing theories based on the principle of starvation and the avoidance of fats, I should have been known all over the countryside as "Fatty" —despite my output of physical energy. No amount of exercise should have been able to offset the diet on which I thrived. Also, according to these theories I should have made a good start towards all the ailments that have been attributed to cholesterol—though, of course, that word wasn't in our vocabulary then. Today, cholesterol gets a good deal more concern than it deserves.

It was in 1923 with this fresh-pork regimen well behind me and my medical career just beginning, that a 16-year-old boy who lay in a diabetic coma was given into my care. Quite probably the lad was turned over to a doctor of unimpressive experience because the patient was going to die anyway, so how could it matter.

In those days, any diabetic under 25 years old was considered a hopeless case. To be sure, insulin was by then being heard of in medical circles. I had read about insulin in some medical journal. But except at the University of Toronto, no one had actually seen insulin, much less employed that drug in diabetes. Toronto University was far out ahead in research in diabetes because Dr. Frederick Banting and Dr. Charles Best, who had discovered the relationship of insulin to diabetes control, were associated with that seat of learning.

In my youthful innocence I didn't realize the presumption in my act when I wrote to Dr. Banting asking whether he could provide me with the insulin which I hoped might save my patient. A Dr. Campbell replied for Dr. Banting. He told me there was only about a tablespoon of the drug in existence. Granting my request was out of the question.

By then, I had made the saving of that stricken boy a dedication. He was a fine lad; one who deserved to live. The best I had been able to do, however, was to bring him out of the coma. Nothing, it seemed to me, would preserve his life so long as his system was utilizing only half of his sugar intake— the little quantity of sugar a patient is given in a diabetic diet.

Through all this, I had been reading every medical writer who might offer anything touching on my problem: Joslyn, Newberg, Marsh, Sippy, Alverez, and Von Norden. From Von Norden, a "high-fat man," I derived an idea which reinforced the memory of my pork-fed boyhood.

I prescribed pork chops for my patient—fat ones, and plenty of them, *three times a day!* It was unheard of. My colleagues contended I was dooming the boy to an even earlier death. If so, then so be it. He was going to die anyhow, according to everything medicine then knew. Why should he have to die hungry?

But he did *not* die! In three days, his urine was sugar-free. If Von Norden was a "high-fat man," young Dr. Reinsh had joined his school with a vengeance.

What I had done was to call on the boy's digestive furnace to burn more fiercely by providing his body with plenty of fuel for its fire. This fatty fuel had burned away the sugar— just as my youthful stuffing of myself with fresh pork had burned away whatever obesity-makers I had consumed, and had burned them away without leaving any bulky residue from the fuel. It was but a short step to arrive at my conviction that plenty of fat meat could play a prominent role in controlling obesity.

Back in those days when a patient came into a doctor's office to ask what could be done about his weight, he generally wanted to put more pounds on a scrawny physique. Medicine has recognized that the overly-skinny individual burns up his food too completely. The problem—not often satisfactorily resolved—is to dampen the furnace by setting the thermostat lower. We doctors call this controlling an over-active metabolism.

It is inescapable logic that the obese person requires exactly the opposite treatment; his thermostat must be set *higher*. The fat person's furnace should consume at a greater rate; and particularly, his body should be made to burn up more starch. It is equally obvious that the fat person's starch intake must be radically reduced: there should be no piling in of the stuff that he will be at pains to incinerate.

Not long ago, the press wires carried the account of a United States Navy medical team's experiments directed, among other things, at discovering exactly what happens when a person undergoes starvation. A group of men were put on the extreme diet of no food at all—just water.

What the Navy researchers found must have proved unsettling to those theorists who persist in telling us that cutting down calories is the way to get rid of the unwanted part of a human body's weight.

Of course, deprivation of all food accomplished a rapid weight loss. The subjects of the experiments lost an average of 20 pounds in ten days. That part of the outcome was predictable enough.

But the theorists were jolted when they learned just *where* the weight was lost. Sixty-five percent of the loss was contributed by the lean tissues; only 35 percent by fat—or by my diagnosis, starch. In fact, the ratio of fat to the total body weight increased by a percentage point. Mainly, as you see, it was the stuff of which sturdiness is made that disappeared; the blubber was far less affected. The Associated Press quoted Lieutenant Commander Fred L. Benoit on this aspect of the tests after he had described them to the American College of Physicians. The Lieutenant Commander said, "Although clinically desirable weight reduction occurs during fasting, it is at the expense of lean tissue—which is physiologically undesirable."

But starvation was not the only method of weight reduction which the Navy men tried. Some subjects were also put on a high-fat, low-calorie diet. Among this group, the average weight loss was only 13 pounds in ten days. However—and this is a big however—only three percent of the loss was contributed by the lean tissues. Fat accounted for 97 percent of the reduction.

These findings didn't amaze me in the slightest, for I had been working on the metabolic thermostat approach to obesity control for years. As for those who may still have trouble believing these facts, I ask them to recollect pictures they've seen of the victims of starvation. Though the figure has become scarcely more than a skeleton, the paunchy abdomen remains—a bulging protuberance but little altered after nearly all else has been consumed by a body that has been cannibalizing itself. Why? Because there was insufficient fuel for the digestive furnace to burn that starch away.

Pause to consider the Eskimos. Few of them would be able to crawl in and out of their igloos if eating fat made its eaters fat. They exist on a diet of meat and blubber. That that diet fails to make them obese was one of the significant observations made by Vilhjalmur Stefansson, the famed explorer of the Arctic who spent long periods living among the Eskimo.

It seemed incredible to Stefansson that a folk could exist from infancy to old age on a diet that was virtually 100 percent fat and protein. Yet there was no gainsaying the evidence. Later, Stefansson's researches at New York's Bellevue Hospital confirmed the virtues of the Eskimo eating habits. His studies of fat as a dietary staple crystallized my confidence in what I had already surmised to be the proper approach to obesity control.

The nomadic Indians who summer on the shores of James Bay engage in setting trap lines in winter and shooting geese in summer. They subsist on what they bag, eating meat and fish almost exclusively. Yet they are stalwart physical specimens, and they never ever heard of cholesterol.

Far from there being anything deleterious about fatty meat, it is one of the safest foods a person can take into his system. An ideal fuel for the body's furnace, it builds sturdiness while taking off the unwanted poundage of excess starch and waterlogging.

Starchy foods and carbohydrates do the exact reverse, and are the worst things a person with a tendency toward obesity can include in his menu. This is not an astounding revelation. Anyone who has inquired at all about dietary practices is aware that Americans consume starchy food in excessive quantity. The panting, discontented people who come to me seldom fail to realize that indulgence in starchy food is the arch fiend responsible for their bulk. But they cannot go without eating. And they mistakenly assume that, bad as starch is for them, fats would be even worse.

The cholesterol scare is doubtless responsible for much of this misconception—a scare which has arisen out of fallacious theories. Those of us who minister to fat people know how wrong the "cholesterol people" have been in their conclusions. We prove their error every day.

The foods I recommend are essential to your well-being. They will not hurt you in any way. They aren't going to harden your arteries. They will not give you arteriosclerosis. And you can forget about the bogeyman cholesterol.

Those who comprehend arteriosclerosis know that what hardens arteries is nicotine and tension. If your furnace is fired up as it should be, cholesterol and all the other clinkers in your system, will be burned up. To use the medical term, your unwanted starches will be metabolized.

What the obese person needs is to replace his starch with protein cells. How to do this? Here's how.

When the food intake is 80 percent protein and fats, the body's thermostat is pushed up. Now the fats burn the starch away, and the starch is replaced by compact, firm healthy protein tissues. Moreover, as the fatty fuel in the body's furnace burns away the bulky carbohydrates, they too, become contributors to the heat and energy. Yes, indeed, fats are the right fuel for the human furnace!

The process induced by the ingestion of fats proceeds at a measured rate which permits the skin to shrink and fit the smaller, firmer body. The patient is not left with the appearance of having recently recovered from some debilitating illness.

In the diet I recommend, no harm will result to your system through malnutrition. The foods upon which you will live will be properly balanced, and will afford sufficient bulk so that you achieve satiety.

In obesity control, the details of treatment must be tailored to the individual. Human systems vary, and these variables can best be discerned by a physician. Each individual's idiosyncracies must be taken into account.

Forget about the generalized rot you hear from the faddist, the masseur, the steam-room attendant, or from your Aunt Tilly. Too many people hover around the fringes of medicine. Ask yourself how much research any of these people have really done.

In obesity control, correct methods call for some of the organs to work harder than they have been doing. This is imperative. These organs have failed to do their job fully. They have lazily put aside some of what you have eaten, and this excess intake has accumulated in the form of so-called fat.

Just to give you an idea of the kind of diet with which I have succeeded: dinner calls for a plentiful serving of meat, fish, or fowl, along with whatever fats happen to be in or on those foods; two or three cooked vegetables with plenty of cream or butter; followed by coffee, tea, or milk. Almost all desserts are forbidden; but on the other hand, you can eat to satiety; there is no ban on second helpings.

The word "diet" has become a dirty word. There is no need for that to be so; one must just eat wisely.

Obesity
Can Be Corrected

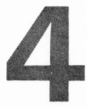

MY PERSONAL INTEREST in obesity as a medical problem has persisted through nearly 40 years as a physician and surgeon. My conclusions are drawn from a lifetime of observations of fat people, and from the breadth of my clinical experience in treating those people. The dimension of this experience is indicated by my case load, which I keep consistently at 450 patients monthly. I have to put a limit on the number of patients I can adequately care for, and I have a waiting list whose most recently added name can't be called for nearly a year.

I am not alleging that that many patients pass through my

office at closely spaced intervals. If they did, none could have the time with me which is a patient's due. Early in the treatment the patient does have a fairly frequent appointment schedule. But after he has progressed, the patient comes in only for an occasional check-up, much the same as any prudent person with any other correctable and controllable disease would.

My patients find that soon enough their clothes will become frightfully loose; even their shoes become too big. If you stick to my diet, you might even have to have your bowling ball redrilled. They look in the mirror, and find that early in the process a smooth transition is apparent. The effect carries to all parts of the body. Of course, the scale yields a more accurate computation of the percentage of weight loss.

My records reveal a wide range of weight loss. The greatest was 148½ pounds; the smallest, 26 pounds. The former represents a weight reduction of more than 47 percent; the 26 pounds was about 17 percent. I once had a patient, who under my treatment shed 39½ pounds between July and October.

The patient who holds the record for me was a 55-year-old woman who weighed 310 when she came to me for treatment. The last entry on her card shows her weighing 161¾. This loss required almost two years. My notation on her cards says: "Claims she holds a new lease on life."

One of my other cards reads: "Plenty rough going. Will not give up. But I am sure she will lose 40 more before leveling off."

It is not always steady progress for the patient who is in treatment for obesity, no more than the victim of any disease always achieves a steady improvement. The woman who wouldn't give up had already lost 83½ pounds from the 265 she started out with. That took 30 months of treatment.

One month saw no progress at all. Worse still, during one two-month period, she actually backslid by half a pound. Some of the less determined, however, undergo periods of backsliding which are far more discouraging than this lady's.

I recall two particular cases when progress seemed to stop for a while. In one of these cases, my card reads: "Romance has interfered with regular eating and drinking habits."

The other card says: "Typical business man. Holiday entertaining has slowed his progress." Ah well, into each life some distractions are bound to fall.

But the satisfactions which come from strict adherence to the control program are more than amply rewarding. These satisfactions are great enough, in most cases, to stay the enticements which the patient knows are his poison. These enormous satisfactions shine through in the statements made by patients recorded in my files.

Some of my records are complete, ending with the attainment of the goal; others show the state of progress in mid-career; others tell of drop-outs and incorrigible backsliders. These records illustrate why I said at the beginning that obesity can be controlled without discomfort or inconvenience, but cannot be completely cured. It is always latent, and ready to assail those who think they can eat and drink absolutely as they please, once a certain weight level has been reached.

By far the greater number of my patients have been women. Men are no less subject to obesity than women, but men do much more talking than acting when it comes to ridding themselves of starch and waterlogging. This is one of the reasons, I am sure, why there are many more widows than widowers.

Make no mistake about it, obesity *is* correctable. You may not have noticed, but nowhere have I spoken of curing it. The obesity-control drop-out will, in a very short time, be right back at his former weight. *Let no one tell you that there is any method of weight reduction which, having succeeded, will remain a success without faithful observance of the regimen which brought about the poundage decrease.*

THAT IS WHY OBESITY CONTROL MUST BE A REGIMEN THE PATIENT CAN LIVE WITH HAPPILY FOR THE REST OF HIS LIFE.

Obesity control requires a prescribed diet. Its specifics will be gone into in the next chapter. For the present, let it merely be said that "a proper diet" is not a synonym for starvation, nor for eternal sameness of food intake. The victim of obesity can eat well and still keep his disease under control.

Starch, which can be burned away when the digestive furnace is fueled with generous amounts of the proper foods, has a peculiar resistance to under-nourishment. Sinews shrivel; organs begin to malfunction. Flesh disappears, and the skin hangs in folds. The weakened system becomes a veritable magnet for disease and infection. But the starchy deposits—the accumulations represented by the paunchy stomach—remain even unto death.

The Diet You Can
Stay on a Lifetime

LET US THINK of the digestive system as a furnace which is controlled by a thermostat. When the furnace's fire is burning so low that it is not consuming all of your nourishment intake, two things need doing. One, the thermostat's setting must be raised; and two, the quality of the fuel must be improved.

When these two matters have been taken care of, the furnace will burn much more hotly, incinerating the body's excess starch. *Waterlogged starch*—the starch the body could not utilize—is, I contend, a much more precise word than fat for describing the substance of obesity.

Proper fuel is what basically does the job. The digestive

organs are not going to be made to work harder if they are fueled skimpily with flaccid foods. Your organs can be revved up to work harder—only if they are plentifully fed with substantial food of the right kinds. And these foods happen to be enormously appetizing and tasteful.

Grant that bread and desserts, of which you may be very fond, are among the items forbidden. Obviously, more starch should not be supplied when there is already too much starch present. But surely it is no hardship to make up for the absence of bread with a second helping of pork chops, pot roast, or roast beef. And if you like your meat succulently fat, then so much the better.

Proteins and fats will be increased to constitute 80 percent of your diet; starches will be cut to 20 percent or less. The thermostat has been pushed up, and away we go. You are now embarked on an uncomplicated, but effective way, to become thinner.

Fat is the master key to obesity control! In its fundamentals, the plan of eating I recommend is the same diet I would order for an athlete. You, the patient, must eat meats, fats, oils, vegetables, and only a limited quantity of fruit. You must also eat three good meals a day. You can hit into snacks when the right kind are available, and when meals are too far apart for your personal comfort.

In almost every kind of treatment, there must, of course, be DON'TS as well as DO'S, so right at the outset let us dispose of the subject of what not to eat.

FORBIDDEN

1. **No flour products.** No bread, cakes, pies, pastries, cookies, macaroni, spaghetti, noodles, or pizza of any kind. Also no cornstarch, soy flour, or cornmeal.

2. **No potatoes.**

3. **No cereals.** This rules out barley, bran, oatmeal, farina, rice, hominy, Corn Flakes, Krispies, Shredded Wheat, Puffed Rice, wheat germ, Krumbles, Post Toasties, Wheatena, Corn Grits, low-calorie cereals, or what have you.

4. **No ice cream.**

5. **No candy.**

6. **No soft drinks of any kind.** This prohibition embraces low-caloried drinks.

7. **No apples.** No applesauce, no baked apples.

8. **No highly salted foods.** (such as anchovies).

In addition to these eight prohibited categories, the following foods are restricted: beans, lentils, corn, liquor, nuts, artificial jellos, gelatine, coffee, and liquids in general. More about these later.

COME AND GET IT

1. **All meats no matter how fatty.** Smoked meats, corned beef, pot roast, ham, pork, veal, pastrami, spareribs, sausage, frankfurters, liver, duck, chicken, luncheon meats, bacon, etc. are all O.K.

2. **All fish and seafood.**

3. **Butter, lard, oleomargarine, oil.**

4. **Cream.**

5. **Salad dressings.** This includes mayonnaise.

6. **All vegetables** except potatoes.

Forget all the hogwash you have been told about there being a connection between overweight and the eating of fatty foods. There just isn't any! In fact, meat and its fat—lots of fat—are a primary diet requirement if obesity is to be controlled.

Your Fluid Intake

FLUIDS ARE A PROBLEM for the dieter. Most overweight people are appreciably waterlogged; adding fluid is no way to alleviate the difficulty. Nevertheless, both at table and between meals, there indeed has to be some fluid intake. But you must stay within the limit of a quart-and-a-half daily maximum of fluids, breakfast juices included. You simply must learn to ration yourself to six glasses of fluids a day. By glasses, I mean the eight-ounce kind—not the extra tall ones bartenders keep on hand for so-called long drinks. Those who carry an especially high poundage—say above 250—will probably need two glasses of beverage beyond the prescribed limit.

You must bear in mind that a second cup of coffee at breakfast may forbid a trip to the water cooler later on. Also, you must consider that that second cup at breakfast will consume your entire coffee allotment for the day. For only two cups of coffee per day are permitted, because coffee stimulates the nervous system and augments the stomach's flow of acid. And acid in the stomach creates an inordinate craving for food.

Milk or buttermilk may comprise up to two cups of the daily fluid intake. The rest of the fluid intake should be tea or water. Under no circumstances, soda pop.

It is my contention that carbonated drinks have an especially pronounced waterlogging effect. This has nothing to do with their caloric count. All carbonated beverages create a watery volume which tends to stay stored up in the system. Clinical experience has provided me with plenty of proof that the overweight should avoid soft drinks entirely.

I once had a patient who allowed himself just one rum-and-cola drink every day, and he wound up afflicted with elephant legs. After four weeks of this, I insisted that he take his rum straight. After he followed my advice, no edema ensued. (Edema is a swelling induced by an effusion of watery fluid from the blood vessels into the tissues and intercellular spaces.) The visible effect of edema is the same as just being plain fat.

Then there was the woman who had to remain on my waiting list for six months. A couple of months before her turn came to begin treatment, a friend of hers had a brainstorm and suggested to her that she start her dieting by filling herself every day with low calorie sodas. When she began drinking the stuff she weighed 27 pounds less than the 336 pounds which showed on the scales on her first visit to my office. I have found that one-calorie pop can put from 10 to 15 pounds on a person in a month.

Occasions for making an exception to the quart-and-a-half rule will arise. In exceptionally hot weather, the body will require some increase in the fluid intake. When the heat is excessive, you may increase your fluid intake by two glasses of water per day.

But to best combat the thirst of torrid days, keep a pitcher of good strong tea in the refrigerator. Drink it sparingly at refrigerator temperature, with neither sugar nor lemon added. A few swallows will do wonders for a thirst.

Six glasses of liquid a day may seem to be a very hard regimen to follow. Probably at the start of your diet, it may prove to be an ordeal; but you'll get used to it, and as your weight starts to drop, your gratification will help to alleviate your thirst.

7

Breakfast

I DON'T BELIEVE in skimpy breakfasts. On the contrary, I recommend a good, hearty, satisfying meal to begin the day.

As a starter, you may desire a juice. The breakfast juice must be vegetable only. Orange juice, grapefruit juice, apple juice or any other juice is not allowed. Should you want a change from vegetable juices, a few ounces of the milkman's half-and-half, will be fine.

Your morning drink won't have to be counted into the amount of liquid permitted daily. But more about that later.

Conventional breakfast foods against which there is a firm mandate are, of course, muffins, biscuits, cereals, and other starchy items, such as waffles or wheatcakes.

Meat, of course, has to be a breakfast staple. This may mean a more hearty breakfast than you have been accustomed to. But you'll become accustomed to eating meat at breakfast, and you'll like it. You can choose steak, liver, cutlets, kidneys, lamb chops, or anything else in the meat department.

Eggs are fine for the person determined to burn away starch. The yolk of the egg is fat; the white is protein. How your eggs are prepared is immaterial. They can be fried, scrambled, poached, boiled, or made into an omelet. If you want a change, breakfast eggs may even be deviled with mayonnaise, which will only add more of what's good for you.

Furthermore, you can have eggs in any style you wish, and as many as you want. I suggest a big, luscious omelet fried in butter and accompanied by pork sausage. These little wienies are succulent and they are good for you.

Nor is there any reason in the world why you shouldn't open a can of salmon or a can of tuna or a tin of sardines, or why you shouldn't treat yourself to some unsalty Nova Scotia lox and cream cheese. But what you must be sure of is that the lox and cheese do not rest on a bagel.

Your breakfast will be composed mainly of high-protein foods. When you get up from the table, you will feel satisfied. Furthermore, you will feel satisfied and comfortable throughout the entire day. You will be amazed to find that the craving which you generally experience during the morning for a snack just about disappears.

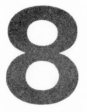

Lunch

YOUR LUNCH should be substantial, too. This is most important in balancing your dietary needs.

Lunch should be eaten at a regular time. Don't let the impulse to do "one more thing" interfere with this regularity. If you have trouble remembering to eat at midday, I recommend that you get yourself an alarm clock to make absolutely certain that you eat on time. For, by delaying your proper time to eat, you work havoc with your appetite. Your craving may become overpowering, and when you ravenously sit down at the table, you are likely to wolf down your food and devour anything and everything. Losing control is not a good thing for the serious weight-reducer.

For lunch, you can make a choice among tuna, boiled ham, salmon, lobster, crabmeat, shrimp, chicken, turkey, hamburger, or broiled fish. If you choose any of the seafoods, you can add as much salad dressing as your heart desires. Since all dressings contain some oil, dressings are good for what ails you. You can, if you so desire, douse your food with plenty of butter or cream.

Some of the recommended items will invariably be found on the luncheon menu of any restaurant. Eat plenty of these foods. You must not feel hunger toward the end of the work-day. Don't try to make do until dinner with snacks. The snacks to be had at an office or in a coffee shop are seldom the sort which overweight people should have. Moreover, late afternoon hunger is likely to lead to increasd fluid intake —an especially disastrous increase when the fluid comes from a soft-drink dispensing machine.

You will not have eaten adequately at noon if you try to make a meal of a tossed salad or of a dish of cottage cheese with fruit. Cheese is something the obesity-control patient may eat, providing he is moderate about it. The reason for this is that cheese has properties which cause the body to retain water. A salad or some cheese is all right along with dinner; but then, at dinner, salads and cheeses are only auxiliaries to the main course.

How about dessert? The answer is no. Have your day's second cup of coffee; or better still, your tea. You can use lemon, and you can sweeten your coffee or your tea if you so desire with an artificial sweetener. If you drink coffee, you can use as much cream as you desire.

Again, remember that lunch never consists of a sandwich simply because breads are irrevocably out. But if you pile up

your plate with tuna, salmon, lobster, or chicken, you'll have
more than plenty to eat.

Dinner

WITH TWO FILLING MEALS under his belt, the person fighting obesity won't be starving mad when he comes to the dinner table. But he must make it a point to eat heartily, nevertheless.

At dinner, meat, fish, and fowl lead the parade. You can have pork, lamb chops, leg of lamb, spareribs, steak, roast beef, roast pork, liver and bacon, ground meats, chicken, turkey, duck, goose—whatever dish your fancy dictates. The servings should be plentiful, and there is no stricture against seconds.

Accompanying the fatty meats should be cooked vegetables, and on the vegetables there should be plenty of butter, margarine, or cream. Like salad dressings, these fats make for tastiness and are great for keeping the fuel stoked high.

To satisfy an insistent sweet tooth and fill the void which some dieters feel when there is no dessert at all, keep a pint of sherbet in the refrigerator. A modest portion of sherbet will assuage the craving for sweetness. A little of it will do less harm than a constant sense of deprivation. Mind, I said a little. What is *a little?* I'd say three tablespoons full at the most.

How about jello? Jello is supposed to be largely a protein food. It is. However, ordinary commercial jello contains a good deal of sugar; and for our weight reducing program, jello would be off limits.

But, then, there is a fairly modern product called D-Zerta. This is a sugarless jello, and therefore should be beyond objection. (There are a number of other products on the market similar to D-Zerta made by other firms.)

During World War I, chemists concocted a gelatin preparation which was specifically used to hold fluids in the body. It was used in emergencies when a soldier, injured in combat, did not have ready access to blood plasma.

In other words, gelatin has the capacity to hold fluids in the system. It is for that reason that I tell my patients that they must go slow on sugarless gelatin products.

Aspics are delicious and consomme madrilene may be a great temptation, but your diet will be far better served if you restrict these delicious dishes to just one a week. Of course, that restriction applies to D-Zerta, and to any other such dessert products.

In Between Meal Snacks

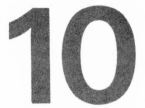

10

LATE AT NIGHT, you may suffer the temptation to eat more. For some compulsive eaters, eating something late at night is a prime necessity. Without that snack, they get fidgety and even ornery suffering anxiety from their deprivation, they can't even fall asleep.

If you must munch something before bedtime, or at any other time for that matter, see that your refrigerator is stocked with an assortment of cold cuts, cocktail sausages, and sardines. These should safeguard you against the temptation to nibble at the sweet and the starchy. No crackers nor toast— no matter how tiny the bite.

How about fruits? Well, for one thing, apples are out entirely. It is my belief that apples operate to cause weight increase.

Some of you may remember the campaign slogan.

> *"An apple a day*
> *Keeps the doctor away!"*

I certainly would not go that far, but I know that if you have a tendency towards obesity, an apple a day wll keep you fat. During World War II, chemists worked up an extract from apples called pectin. Pectin served to hold fluids in the body or men injured in combat, when blood plasma was not immediately available. The implications are clear. I can tell you from long personal observation that I have found it almost impossible to bring down the weight of anyone who keeps on eating apples.

I'd much rather see you eat a banana (which is far starchier than an apple) because bananas do not have the adverse characteristics of apples. As for oranges, grapefruit, and other citrus fruits, I'm sorry but they're definitely out.

How about Alcohol?

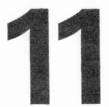

11

For obesity-control patients accustomed to cocktails or beer, there need not be a complete cutoff. You may have a social drink of hard liquor every day, or down a glass of beer, or imbibe a glass of wine.

Steer clear of sweet liqueurs, such as Creme de Menthe, Apricot Brandy, Vermouth, Dubonnet, Curacoa, Sloe Gin, etc; and avoid sweet wines such as Sherry, Port, and Tokay. Champagne is fine. So are the Burgundies, the Sauternes and similar white table wines.

Or you can have a shot of Bourbon, Scotch, Rye, Gin, or Vodka. But keep it to *one* shot. If you add water to your Scotch that must be counted into your daily fluid intake. Of course, club soda is out. The same goes for Quinine Water or Tonic.

For most of us, a drink a day will lift the spirit. This is important for the dieter, who doing without his accustomed pies, cakes, breads, potatoes, and candies may feel deprived. But remember that whatever the preference, alcoholic drinks must be held to an absolute ceiling of seven a week. The dieter should, for the most part, ration himself to a one-a-day basis.

However, if a special occasion arises, such as a wedding or a birthday party, and you feel impelled to lift the lid and go for three shots of booze, you can do this provided you make up for your delinquency by laying off the stuff for the next two days. Alternately, you can skip your daily alcoholic allotment for two or three days prior to the anticipated celebration, and thus pile up credits to be expended when the festive evening rolls around. This last method of rationing is by far the best, psychologically. For it is much easier to do without a drink when you know that you're going to enjoy a gala night a few days hence, than it is to repentantly forego the drink you want with no special whoopee to look forward to.

If a patient of mine is not showing satisfactory progress and I ascertain that his lack of result is due to cheating on alcohol, I put the sauce altogether off limits for him. This is not a punishment; it's a protection.

Forbidden Foods

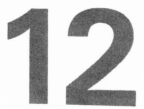

IF YOU ARE A PERSON who sincerely wants to be rid of the blubbery starch which is so disquieting when you step on the bathroom scale, and if you are seriously determined that your excess avoirdupois shall not return once it has disappeared, you must rigidly keep to the rules. Half measures won't do. There are certain foods you just can't eat! For *your* system, they're just plain poison.

You must maintain strict self-discipline both when you sit down to eat your meals, and when you go prowling through the refrigerator for between-meal snacks. There will be plenty of good things you may eat at both times—but there are some stern *Don'ts*. Here they are:

1. *No bread in any form, size, or shape.* This means no rolls, no muffins, no biscuits, no toast, no diet breads, no crackers, no bagels, no pumpernickel, no bialys. Bread and its counterparts are banned *totally!*

   Bread bloats the stomach. Bread is so very starchy it creates a craving for fluids, and bread therefore rates as an indirect cause of waterlogging.

   There is one thing I know about bread which has been taught me by experience: When a patient stops eating bread, he experiences a new comfort.

   If a patient of mine refuses to leave bread alone, there is nothing I can do to help him, and we may as well call it quits. He is dropped fast so that his place may go to a more seriously intentioned fighter against obesity.

2. *No flour.* This excludes whole wheat flour, the so-called health flours like rice flour, soy bean flour, cornstarch, cornmeal, etc. All flours are banned.

   Flour will come sneaking your way in various forms, like in those famous French sauces—Bechamel or Mornay—or flour will be an integral part of dishes such as Southern-fried Chicken. Avoid this trap.

   However, if your hostess serves pot roast which contains two tablespoonsful of flour for thickening, and the dish has been prepared for 10 persons, your share of the flour is so mighty little you don't have to make a Federal case out of it. Common sense will tell you in most situations what you can cut and what you can't.

3. *A limit of three fruits per week.* Most fruits contain excessive amounts of carbohydrate. That is why I permit

only bananas, peaches, and pears. And each of the permitted fruits may be eaten only once a week.

Canned pears and canned peaches are out; they contain excess sugar. However, if nothing else is available, pour off every drop of the syrup, and you won't be doing too much harm.

Slice the bananas and add milk or cream, or douse them in a salad dressing.

Never eat cottage cheese with fruit, for the cheese causes the body to hold water. Remember how boiled skim milk used to be used to stop diarrhea? Cottage cheese does the same thing.

4. *No fruit juices.* This may be a blow, but you will have to sustain it. And don't worry about your vitamin intake. There are other sources of vitamins besides orange juice, and you will be getting plenty. Besides, you can always buy your vitamins and take them straight out of a bottle.

5. *No salt on your food.* Salt is well known for its ability to cause the storage of fluids in the body. That is why salt tablets are used in extremely hot weather to prevent heat prostration.

So keep the salt-cellar off the table till you've broken yourself of the habit. Many people just shake salt on their food as an unconscious action; it is somewhat like a reflexive response to having a dish placed in front of them. But this a reflex the obese can't afford. Make it a point to use salt only in preparation of foods.

As a substitute for salt, you can use almost any kind of herbs or vinegar. Try sprinkling some chopped parsley on your food or some fresh basil. Experiment, and you will be surprised what taste vistas open.

Steer clear of green olives, cole slaw, and dill pickles. Banish lox, and other highly piquant smoked fish such as anchovies, which you know are loaded with salt.

6. *A maximum of six cups of liquid per day*. (See Chapter 6)

7. *No sugars or starches.*

8. *A severe restriction on beans, corn, and lentils*. These are allowed in highly moderated amounts once a week, and only for the sake of variety. Your ration is one ear of corn a week; one half-cup of beans; and one half-cup of lentils. Don't go overboard here or your waistline will show it.

9. *A limit of one alcoholic drink per day*. This drink can be wine, or almost any hard liquor. Restrict beer to one eight-ounce glass a week. (See Chapter 11).

10. *No carbonated beverages*. (See Chapter 11)

11. *Severely limit your intake of nuts*. Nuts are a high-protein food; but nuts are insidious. You can sit and nibble them hour after hour, and without realizing it, eat so many nuts that they will be quite the equivalent of a full day's meals. So that nuts do not get the better of you, I restrict your intake to a maximum of 12 nuts a day,

and I restrict your peanut butter to one-half teaspoonful per day.

There is nothing essentially wrong about including nuts in your diet. The oil content is beneficial. But it is so easy to overindulge that precautions must be taken.

And, of course, salted nuts are out entirely.

*   *   *

How about Chinese cooking? Well, if you must, but only on occasion and then sparingly. Most Chinese dishes contain gobs of corn starch.

Practically all Chinese foods are fried in oil, and that makes them good for you. But that cornstarch—that's a different matter!

However, you can have a few spareribs occasionally, remembering that Chinese ribs are invariably marinated in honey, a forbidden food. Best to stick to the roast pork, avoiding the so-called duck sauce—in reality a plum sauce—which is definitely off limits.

But no noodles, no rice, no preserved fruits. If you keep to seafood, duck, chicken, pork, lobster, and beef for the most part, your excursion to Chinatown won't be so expensive, dietarily speaking.

Above all, be very sparing with that gravy that comes with *Eggs Foo Yung;* that gravy is loaded with starch. So, too, is the golden crust on egg-rolls. If you must—sort of once in a blue moon—and as a pure concession—eat half of one egg-roll, no more.

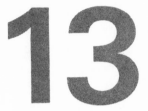

13

Your Diet Dictionary

IN MY LONG EXPERIENCE in obesity control, I have found that, again and again, patients ask me questions such as: "May I eat this?" or "May I eat that?" In order that there may be no equivocation or doubt, I am setting forth specifics about just every food that I can think of. If you go on the diet I recommend, the following list should become your Bible.

Ale   Yes. One glass per week. Counts the same as any other alcoholic beverage. You can swig a full eight-ounce glass.

Almonds	All right if you limit them to 12 a day and you don't eat any other kind of nuts during that period.
Anchovies	Very salty. Omit.
Apples	No!
Apple juice	Out.
Applesauce	Forbidden.
Apricots	Leave them alone.
Apricot juice	Not for you.
Artichokes	Why not!
Asparagus	All you care to eat.
Avocado	O.K.
Bacon	Right up our alley.
Bamboo Shoots	No harm here.
Bananas	One a week.
Barley	Definitely no. This is a very fattening, starchy cereal.
Basil	Yes.
Beans	One-half cupful a week.
Beef	Pile it on.
Beef Stew	No objection if it doesn't contain potatoes.
Bechamel Sauce	No, made with flour.
Beer	One eight-ounce glass permitted once a week.
Beets	Yes.
Benedictine	Steer clear of this one. It's loaded with sugar.
Biscuits	Keep a mile away.
Blackberries	Forbidden.
Blueberries	Deny yourself.

Blue Cheese	O.K.
Bologna	Fine.
Bouillabaisse	Oil, seafood, and vegetables — all on the permitted list.
Bouillon	Whether in commercial cubes or made from beef or chicken, O.K.
Bran	A three-star No.
Brandy	Just one on any day.
Brazil Nuts	Go very slow here.
Bread	Strictly out the window—whether it's white bread, brown bread, black bread, corn bread, Vienna bread, French bread, Italian bread, or bread made with enriched flour. Even if the bread is made by the gods themselves, the answer is clearly no.
Brie Cheese	O.K.
Broccoli	Yes.
Brown Sauce	No, no! Made with flour.
Brussels Sprouts	Yes.
Buckwheat	No.
Buns	No, No, No.
Burgundy	O.K. but restrict to six ounces per day.
Butter	All you want.
Butternuts	Handle with care.
Buttermilk	Yes.
Cabbage	In any form you desire.
Cake	All and every variety are completely off limits.
Camembert	O.K.
Candy	Of no kind or variety.

Cantaloupe	No.
Carbonated beverages	Definitely no. It doesn't make any difference if the bottle is high-calorie, low calorie or just plain soda water.
Carrots	O.K.
Cashews	O.K. but limited to a dozen a day.
Catsup	No, not even if it's spelled Ketchup.
Cauliflower	O.K.
Caviar	Fish eggs in oil. It's your dish.
Celery	Fine!
Chablis	O.K. within the prescribed limit.
Champagne	Six-ounce glassful.
Chard	Yes.
Cheddar Cheese	O.K.
Cherries	No.
Chicken fat	No need to stint.
Chick Peas	See lentils.
Chicken	Fine. All you want, boiled, baked or fried. But no Southern-Fried chicken —too much flour.
Chicory	Yes.
Chili con carne	Those beans are a hazard, but still O.K. once a week, if the portion is restricted to one cupful.
Chili Powder	Yes.
Chili Sauce	No. Too much sugar.
Chives	Yes.
Chocolate	Never.
Chopped Liver	All ingredients are go.
Chutney	Generally filled with sugar. I'd say no.

Cider	An apple derivative. Verboten!
Cinnamon	Yes.
Clams	All you care to eat.
Clam chowder	The potatoes kill it.
Coca Cola	Out.
Cocoa	Never.
Cocomalt	You must be kidding!
Coconut	Steer clear.
Coffee	Fine, but limited to two cups per day. Must be counted within the six-cup beverage limit allowable per day.
Cole Slaw	Generally, loaded with salt. Go easy.
Collards	By all means.
Condensed Milk	No.
Consomme	By all means.
Cordials	No. Too sweet; too much sugar.
Corn	Starchy. As a concession, one ear a week.
Corned Beef	Great!
Corn Flakes	A cereal of purest ray serene. A clear negative.
Corn Syrup	Let's not fool around!
Cottage Cheese	O.K. But not along with fruit. Rather you'd go easy here, anyhow.
Crabs	No need to stint.
Crackers	It doesn't make any difference what package they come in, or how big or how small they are, the answer is still no.
Cranberries	Thumbs down.
Cream	Soak it up. It's good for you. Whether

	it's light cream or heavy cream, soak it up.
Cream Cheese	Why not?
Cream of Wheat	Like all other cereals, no.
Crême de mènthe	Sugar-laden. Not for you.
Crisco	On the permitted list.
Cucumbers	Yes.
Curacao	Full of sugar. Not for you.
Currants	No.
Custard	Terrible!
Dandelion Greens	Yes.
Dates	Loaded with sugar. Lay off.
Diet Cola	No!
Dill Pickles	Very sparingly. High salt content.
Donuts	Plain murder for you. Protect your life and run!
Duck	Yes!
D-Zerta	A commercial product made of gelatine, with no sugar content. But like all other gelatines, this must be restricted to one portion a week.
Edam Cheese	Yes.
Egg Nog	Not as bad as it sounds. The egg, the cream and the brandy are okay, but the sugar ruins the concoction. Say one a year, on Christmas afternoon.
Eggplant	Yes.
Eggs	In any form.
Endive	Yes.
Escarole	O.K.
Evaporated Milk	Avoid.

Farina	A big no.
Fat-free Milk	No.
Figs	Off limits.
Finnan Haddie	Fish is okay, even if it's smoked.
Flour	The arch enemy! No matter in what form this comes, it's still out to murder you. Soy flour, enriched flour, whole wheat flour—keep away.
Frankfurters	Fine. No need to be stingy here.
French Gravies	Almost always prepared with flour.
Fricassee	No, almost always prepared with flour.
Frogs Legs	They're delicious fried in butter. Eat all you want.
Fruit Cocktail	Sorry, but the answer is no.
Garlic	No harm, except perhaps to the breath.
Gelatine	Restricted to one portion a week.
Gin	One jigger per day.
Ginger ale	Out.
Goose	If yours is cooked, by all means eat it.
Gooseberries	Out.
Gorgonzola Cheese	Yes.
Grapes	Forbidden fruit.
Grapefruit	Off limits.
Grapefruit juice	No.
Grape juice	Full of sugar. Avoid.
Grape Nuts	Stay a mile away.
Green peas	O.K. but sparingly. A borderline vegetable.

Grits	No matter of what kind, shape, or consistency, they're not for you.
Gruyère Cheese	O.K.
Guava	No.
Guinea Hen	Great!
Ham	Come and get it. But none of the salty variety.
Hamburger	Yes! Yes! Yes!
Headcheese	Why not?
Herring	Matjas herring, Bismarck herring, Swedish herring, no matter what kind of herring—it's all for you. But when heavily salted, ration yourself severely.
Hickory Nuts	A dozen a day, at the very most.
Hollandaise	Lemon juice, butter, egg yolks—all O.K.
Hominy	An enemy.
Honey	No, no, and again no.
Honeydew Melon	So sorry, but no.
Hot Dogs	We ran across this above labelled as frankfurters but a rose by any other name smells just as sweet.
Ice Cream	One powerful no.
Ice Cream Soda	Aw, go on!
Ice milk	No.
Jams	A big negative!
Jellies	Run, run far away!
Jello	Loaded with sugar! Avoid.
Kale	O.K.
Kidney Beans	Once a week only.
Kohlrabi	O.K.

Krumbles	Bad for you.
Kumquats	As you may have expected, no!
Lamb	Yes. Fine for your full buildup.
Lamb Stew	No objection, if prepared without potatoes or dumplings.
Lard	O.K.
Leek	O.K.
Lemon juice	In moderate amount.
Lemonade	Out.
Lemons	Really off limits, but a slice with your tea won't do damage.
Lentils	A border line case. Restrict to one-half cupful once a week.
Lettuce	O.K.
Liederkranz	O.K.
Lima Beans	One half cupful once a week, but then no corn, nor lentils, nor other beans that week.
Limburger Cheese	O.K. if you can stand the smell.
Limes	Same as lemons.
Liverwurst	By all means.
Lobster	An excellent high-protein food.
Loganberries	No.
Luncheon meat	No restriction.
Macadamia Nuts	Same as Brazil Nuts.
Macaroni	Run a mile! This kind of thing can kill you.
Mangos	No.
Manhattan Cocktail	Yes, but restricted to one a day.
Margarine	Okay.
Marmalade	Beyond your reach.

Marshmallows	Awful!
Martini	Okay, if you hold to one a day.
Matzoth	A resounding nix.
Mayonnaise	All you want. This is primarily a combination of eggs and oil.
Milk	Fine.
Milk Chocolate	*Verboten.*
Mint	Yes.
Molasses	The world's worst.
Muffins	Of course not!
Mulberries	No.
Mushrooms	All you want.
Mustard	Yes.
Mustard Greens	Yes.
Nectarines	Same as peaches.
Noodles	Run for your life.
Noodle Soup	No.
Nutmeg	O.K.
Oatmeal	Nix.
Okra	Yes.
Olives (Green)	No. Too salty.
Olives (Ripe)	Full steam ahead.
Old-fashioned Cocktail	Once a day only.
Omelette	Fine. Combination of eggs and butter.
Onions	Yes.
Orange	No.
Orange Ice	A concession. But restrict to three tablespoonsful, three times a week.
Orange Juice	No.

Oregano	Yes.
Oysters	Why not?
Pancakes	Might as well be spelled P-O-I-S-O-N.
Papaya	No.
Parmesan Cheese	Fine.
Parsley	O.K.
Parsnips	O.K., but go very easy here.
Pastry	Not on your life.
Paté	Liver and oil. Nothing wrong here.
Peaches	A permitted fruit. One a week.
Peanuts	Keep it down to 12 a day at most.
Peanut butter	One teaspoonful a day, as a dessert, when you are not having fruit.
Pears	One a week.
Pecans	Unsalted. And then only a dozen a day at most.
Peppers	O.K.
Pepsi-Cola	Out!
Persimmons	No.
Pie	Never!
Pimento	O.K.
Pineapple (canned)	No.
Pineapple (raw)	Still no.
Pineapple juice	No.
Pistachio Nuts	Limit: 12 a day.
Plantain	No.
Plums	Same as peaches.
Pomegranate	No.
Popcorn	Keep out of sight.

Postum	Okay, but must be limited in accordance with six-cup-daily limitation of liquids.
Potato Chips	Hands off.
Potatoes	Turn away.
Pretzels	Satan in an appealing disguise.
Prune Juice	Avoid.
Prunes	A ruination.
Puddings	A thousand times no.
Pumpkin	O.K.
Rabbit	Fine.
Radishes	Yes.
Raisins	No.
Raspberries	Not for you.
Remoulade Sauce	O.K. Mayonnaise with various herbs.
Rhubarb	O.K. if prepared without sugar, or with artificial sugar.
Rice	A starchy vegetable that can do you no good.
Rolls	No.
Rocquefort Cheese	O.K.
Rum	A jigger once a day.
Rutabagas	Yes.
Salmon	Just what the doctor ordered.
Salt	Avoid. Allowable only in highly restricted amounts.
Sardines	Yes.
Sauterne	O.K. within the prescribed limit.
Scallops	A good high-protein food.
Scotch	Okay, but remember—just one four-

	ounce gulp a day.
Scrapple	Yes.
Sherbet	Only if you must, and then only three tablespoons at the most. Sherbet contains a good deal of sugar. I make this concession because the flesh is weak and some people simply must taste a bit of sweet, or else they just can't make it at all. If you handle this allowance in moderation, you will still get by and do well.
Shish Kebab	Excellent.
Shredded Wheat	Leave it for those who long to be fat.
Shrimp	Splendid.
Soufflée	No, no!
Southern-Fried Chicken	A wolf in sheep's clothing. It's smothered in batter, and batter is flour.
Soy Beans	Once a week. (See lima beans.)
Soy Sauce	O.K.
Spaghetti	You might as well embrace the devil.
Spinach	Yes.
Squash	O.K.
Strawberries	Sorry, no!
Sugar	The devil incarnate. Makes no difference whether the sugar is white, brown, or packed in gold foil.
Sweetbreads	Okay.
Sweet Pickles	No.
Sweet Potatoes	No.

Swiss Cheese	Yes.
Tangarines	No.
Tapioca	A false friend. Loaded with starch.
Tartar Sauce	O.K. Mayonnaise with herbs.
Tea	Fine, but remember that six-cup limitation on liquids.
Thyme	Yes.
Tomatoes	Yes.
Tom Collins	No. This one is made with sugar, and sugar is out for you.
Tomato juice	Yes—breakfast only.
Tomato Soup	No.
Tongue	No restriction here.
Tuna Fish	Excellent.
Turkey	Pile it on.
Turnips	Yes.
Veal	Good for you.
Velouté Sauce	No, made with flour.
Vermouth, French	Count this the same as any other drink.
Vermouth, Italian	On the sweet side. Better not.
Vinegar	O.K.
Waffles	To ask the question is to answer it.
Walnuts	Twelve a day at most.
Watercress	O.K.
Watermelon	No.
Wax beans	O.K.
Wheatena	Thumbs down.
Wheat germ	May be awfully healthy, but not for

	you.
Wheaties	Leave it for the kids.
Whiskey	Okay, provided you keep it to a solo drink each day.
Whitefish	A delicacy that is your privilege.
White Sauce	No! No! Made with flour.
Wine	Keep away from the sweet ones like Port, Muscatel, and Sherry. Red and white table wines are permitted. Hold to six ounces a day.
Worcestershire Sauce	O.K.
Yams	No.
Yeast	O.K.
Yogurt	O.K.

To Help You over the Rough Spots

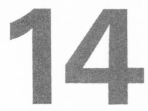

IT IS A CREDO of the business world that policy can best be formulated, decisions reached, and transactions concluded amid the clatter of a restaurant and the repeated intrusions of a confused waiter. Considering American business ways, it is something of a miracle to me that any executive retains a whole stomach and a set of arteries which won't crack in a strong breeze.

For the obesity-control patient who must function in this milieu, the best way out is the white lie. Whether host or guest, he can fabricate a story of some esoteric digestive disorder and of stringent medical strictures which limit him to the luncheon menu I have described, with nothing more potent for drink than coffee or milk.

Why the white lie? Because there is widespread acceptance that disobeying your doctor is unthinkable when there is an actual stomach ailment, whereas on the contrary, doctors who administer diets are old fuddy-duds and killjoys and disobeying "just this once," won't matter so much anyhow. This is particularly so in the matter of drinks. Colleagues press so much less about food than they do about martinis.

True, one martini a day is within the limits of our obesity-control program, but that drink is likely to be much more needed and pleasurable *after* work than in the hurry-flurry of a noontime dining date.

Social occasions also put the obesity-control patient's will power to a hard test. Luncheons, brunches, banquets, receptions, church suppers, company picnics, bridge teas, and all other such gatherings are high hurdles to be cleared.

If you know you hostess well enough, you can tell her the truth in advance, and ask her to prepare for you a plate of what you can eat. If you find such a procedure embarrassing, you can eat before you go; and resorting to the business luncheon white lie, merely nibble at what is set before you. Or you can fill up later at home—after the party—on the meat and vegetables your diet calls for.

Your program should include a record of your weekly weight. You should also start your diet by making a written record of your suit size or your dress size, and of your various body measurements taken in the nude. Chest or breast sizes should be taken at the nipples. The girth of your abdomen should be recorded by the tape measure rolled around your body at the umbilicus. You should also write down your circumferences at the hips, and the thickness of your thighs where they are the largest. Measure your calves, too, and the circumference of your neck. This data constitutes your starting record.

You may juggle the order of your meals to fit your particular circumstances. You can start the day with dinner, then eat lunch, and wind up with breakfast, if that arrangement suits you.

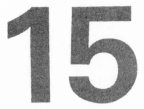

The Need for Exercise

IT IS SAID *ad nauseam* that most Americans who live in our push-button age do not get enough exercise because most people can earn a living without doing physical work. Exercise, we hear, is largely limited to getting in and out of automobiles, which turns out to be highly insufficient despite the acrobatics modern car design requires. True, Americans golf, bowl, dance, ski, and keep riding stables solvent. Transient fads such as the Frug, and perennials such as the Square Dance, are by no means sedentary pastimes. In some degree, these activities compensate for the wholesale disapppearance of the physical work once so generally required to keep a household going. But, by and large, the exercise men and women do is not sufficiently consistent to keep weight down.

Let me emphasize that no diet is worth a tinker's so-and-so unless it is accompanied by a steady program of exercise. This regimen must be followed each and every day, without exception. Your exercise program should be written down by you on paper, in black and white, and carried out diligently. At first, you will find this an ineffable bore. What is more, you may develop aches and pains. The temptation to side-step this chore will be great indeed; but at the risk of being obnoxious, I emphasize that the success of your diet depends on keeping yourself trim and in shape. Physical rehabilitation of the organs of digestion is a *must* if the diet I've outlined is to succeed.

As the pounds roll off, it is up to you to tighten and spruce up your physique. If you do, you will feel like a million dollars. But, let me re-emphasize, that diet alone won't work—you must simultaneously activate your digestive system.

Now I am not proposing that you suddenly become an athlete. Quite the contrary! I am cautioning you to start easy. But the point I stress is that you must *start,* and you must start *immediately*—if your diet is to be effective. The day of confrontation cannot be put off.

If you are over 30 years of age, your exercise program should be tailored to your weight, your age, and your general physical condition. A doctor can be of great assistance here. But if you do not have a coronary condition and if you use your head, you can make up an exercise program for yourself that will not put you in peril.

The first thing to bear in mind is the slogan of the joggers: *Train—Don't strain!* You must condition your body to the exercise it has not had; you can't thrust yourself into a program, and suddenly use muscles that have softened and weakened from disuse. These muscles must gradually—I repeat *gradually*—be brought into use again. A good way to start is to go to your YMCA, or YWCA, or YMHA, or local gymnasium, and sign up for a course, or at least get a little advice. Failing that, you can acquire a copy of the Canadian Air Force Exercise Manual at any bookstore, or you can get a copy of some other such book which lays out a program of gradually increased exercise.

But whatever you do, be guided by this principle: *When you're tired, stop!* Don't force yourself to accomplish feats that are really beyond your powers. I don't mean that you stop exercising the moment you feel uncomfortable. You're *bound* to feel uncomfortable the first few times around. But feeling a little pull in the muscles which yields discomfort is quite a different thing from running your heart to a point of strain.

Let us take the simple exercise called *The Sit-Up*. In this exercise, you lie prone on the floor with your feet, your back, the palms of your hands, and the back of your head touching the floor. Now you raise your body at the trunk, elevating your torso so that it becomes perpendicular to the floor. This exercise is simple enough, and most everyone can accomplish *The Sit-Up* at least once. A good athlete in condition can do an exercise like this 100 times; and the ordinary person can easily work up to a point where he can do 15 or 20 sit-ups without any strain. I might add, though it sounds somewhat unbelievable, that the record is something over 14,000 consecutive sit-ups—which only goes to show what the human body can accomplish through training.

If you're fat and badly overweight, it would be utter folly

for you to try to do more than two sit-ups on your first attempt. As soon as you find that two sit-ups involve no strain, you can go on to three sit-ups, etc. This same principle of gradually increased performance applies to all your calisthenics.

One good way of handling your daily exercises is to choose a guru such as Ed Allen, or Bonnie Pruden, or any one of the other TV people who offer a daily or three-times-a-week program of exercises. Here again, you may find that you can't accomplish everything shown on the screen, or that you can't go along with the full set of exercises. But if you hitch your wagon to some particular star, you will find that your ability to cope will increase day by day. Pretty soon, you'll take part fully.

There are certain exercise gimmicks that you can set up at home. For example, a standard bicycle with a rear type stand can work wonders. If you get on your bike and pedal five or ten minutes twice a day, you'll be putting the old frame into real good shape. Start two hours or so after your last meal, and keep at it till you work up a sweat.

There are also many motorized bikes on the market made especially to serve as exercise machines. These are even better than a regular bicycle, because even when *you* tire, the motored bike keeps going at full pace, and your will to stay with it is thus strengthened.

Just a word here to avoid misunderstanding. There is no need to increase your level of performance, day by day. If you get up to a certain level, you might well maintain that level of performance for a week, or two weeks, or even longer. The muscles then become easily accustomed to that particular level. Then, if you move forward to a new level, you won't suffer undue strain.

Another exercise I recommend is sitting on a chair with your knees spread apart. Then try to bend just enough to nearly touch the floor with the tips of your hands. This exercise puts pressure on the abdomen—and a good healthy pressure it is. In time, you should be able to do the same exercise without any strain at all; and if your weight really comes down, you'll even be placing the palms of your hands flat on the floor.

For men who live in a private house, I recommend getting some heavy cement blocks and putting them in a corner of the basement or in a corner of the garage. Now it may sound dull as dishwater to lift up a heavy cement block, and tote it from one side of the room over to the other side. But there is a certain satisfaction that will come your way when you find that the task, once so arduous, has become a breeze. After a month or two, your performance will stand out as stark, indisputable testimony to the fact that you have built up a set of muscles beyond your fondest hopes.

If you live in the city in an apartment house, you can accomplish more or less the same thing by acquiring a set of barbells. Your first struggles to lift these weights will become a laughable memory after you have practiced with them for two months or so. You will find that your body now contains power you just didn't realize it could muster.

Nevertheless, it is my conviction the very best kind of exercise is the exercise you *enjoy*. And this takes us directly into the realm of sports.

Most sports contain the exhilarating element of competition. For example, bowling itself is a tremendous lot of fun, but outscoring your opponent adds to the zest. The body conditioning you can get from bowling is worthwhile. So get a few friends, and arrange to bowl two or three times a week. As poor as you might do the first time out, I'm sure you'll find one of the party who is in your class or who even does worse. You'll raise a lot of laughs, and the evening out will be fun and relaxation, and certainly not too costly. A few months of this, and you'll find that your score has gone up and up, and that your weight has gone down and down. You'll also find that your skill has improved considerably.

Swimming, while not competitive, is one of the finest exercises you can take. Of course, you can compete with yourself. You may find that the first week you take to the water, even during one lap leaves you breathless. But soon, you'll be doing two laps and then three laps; and after a while, you'll be doing four and five laps, and after your exertion, you'll feel as fresh as a daisy.

One exercise I recommend is to grasp the side of the pool and let your body sink straight down until your back is more or less perpendicular. Then start kicking until your body raises itself to a flat plane. A month or so of this exercise will do wonders for your hips.

Walking is of value, but only if the walking is brisk. If hills are nearby, by all means start to climb them. Get going where the going is rough. Perhaps you can arrange with a few friends to go on regular hikes. Organize a hiking club, if that is possible. It's a great social idea, and it can put your body in good shape.

Golf offers you fresh air, exercise, and relaxation. Relaxation? Did I say *relaxation?* Well, ideally that is what golfing should be, but in all too many cases people become golf nuts and get the idea that they must emulate Arnold Palmer or

Jack Nicklaus. They play every round as if their lives depended upon it. A missed putt becomes the occasion for self-beratement. A pitch over the green brings forth howls of despair. Playing golf in this way produces the anxieties you are trying to get rid of.

Yes, golf is a great game—provided you approach it as *a game*. That is all it is, and that is all it should be, for all of us. Don't try to emulate the professional who spends hours and hours of each day practicing, for that is sheer madness.

Golf can be physically beneficial provided you observe certain rules. To start with, never rent a cart if you can walk. Walk and walk and *walk*—because the exercise is good for you. Secondly, do not stop at those water fountains to drink your fill. That kind of drinking simply makes you *more* thirsty—not less thirsty. Don't patronize the food stands temptingly placed at strategic areas on the course. The food they offer is, for the most part, the wrong kind of food. Wear clothing which will promote perspiration. Perspiring is good for you. And above all, do not eat your heart out every time you make a bad shot. If you insist on acting up this way, you'd be better off to just quit the game entirely.

Horseback riding is excellent.

Tennis is fine, too, but if you are over 35, restrict your tennis to doubles.

The list of sports is too long for me to go into. The main thing to remember is that sports are fine, uplift the spirit, and assist you in acquiring a good figure.

So I say to you go ahead, and put yourself on the diet I have outlined for you, but don't expect results unless you combine your diet with some program of exercise, which you're going to religiously follow each and every day of your life.

The Role
of the Doctor

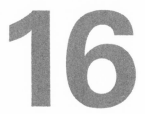

THE TRAGEDY is that the evils of obesity are, in reality, so very great. These evils are not only the discomforts in mind and body and the foregoing of pleasures open to normally proportioned people—the arch evil is that obesity is a shortcut to the grave.

The nature of obesity is controversial. The attempt of science to break down and analyze the body's processes in the utilization of foods tells us next to nothing. We know *what* happens; we do not know *why* these things happen.

It is precisely because obesity is complex that you would be best served in a reduction program to put yourself, if you can possibly manage it, under the care of a doctor. A physician can be helpful in many ways.

I haven't the slightest doubt that you will benefit and make headway if you go it alone on the diet I have prescribed; but your progress and ultimate success will depend on how faithfully you adhere to the tenets of the diet set forth in this book. However, because of unanticipated emotional disturbances, you may, at some future time, falter and be ready to give up your program of weight control. Such disturbances can arise out of family discord, sudden sickness or death in the family, a pile-up in the office, continuous financial worry, and from any other difficulty either real or imagined. Injuries and ailments, too, can undermine your determination to get the better of obesity.

Maybe its your dratted sinus condition, or maybe its your respiratory ailment, or your darned allergy, or your recurrent insomnia, or a wrenched ankle, or a dislocated shoulder, or any painful mishap that can dampen the will to win. Though the illness or injury may seem trivial, the effect of it may easily discombobulate your reducing. In such stress situations, a doctor's counsel can be invaluable. With his help, the day can be saved. If the going gets rough, don't try to go it alone; it may be too much for you.

Certain factors are, of course, so apparent that literate laymen are as aware of them as scientists are. There is, for instance, the decreased physical activity of contemporary life. The effects of sluggishness on the nervous system are manifest and visible. Our way of life is typified by dragging out the family car for a three-block trip to buy a dozen ready-mixed biscuits. Scant exertion results in the manufacture of lots of starch.

Overwork, pressures, apprehensions are our daily lot. The blanketing word for them is "tensions." An etiologist may dispute the reasons, but the fact is that the human animal seeks relief from tensions through eating and drinking. Hence the coffee break, the cocktail hour to unwind, the nightly excursion to the refrigerator.

These attempts at escape and surcease are all contributors to poundage. And since food is sought to allay emotional tumult, the psychological side of obesity cannot be neglected when a weight reduction program is undertaken. Here, again, is one more reason why seeing a doctor is highly advisable when a program of weight reduction is undertaken. There is need for the counsel which his objectivity can provide.

Today, the average American's diet is 80 percent starch. Proteins and fat are on the very short end. In the matter of cost, the starch salesmen have all the better of it. Heavy, starchy filling foods are cheap. But any doctor will tell you that in the cost of good health, you are paying a heavy, heavy price. The body is not a refinery which can change all this starch to fat. Rather, the starch remains in the body just as it entered it—as half-burned clinkers in your furnace.

It is now "old hat" that a fat man is the prime sucker for a heart attack. One need not trot out statistics to show that the fat die much younger than the thin. A person who is afflicted with heart disease is immediately put on a stringent diet by his attending physician. But what the coronary patient needs for a fair chance at survival is a good full diet with a modest amount of salt.

In days past, the elderly almost always died after fracturing a hip. After a misadventure, an old person generally quit eating, and so succumbed to his own unconsumed poisons. Cardiacs can, and do, die similarly when subjected to starvation and to no salt, with a consequent unbalancing of the chemistry of their bodies. I have treated too many cardiacs not to be positive of this. Overweight is something which those afflicted with a heart condition have an especial need to conquer. But for them starvation can be an even shorter cut to the grave than heart failure.

I realize that in putting forward such assertions, I am laying myself open to charges of radicalism if not outright heresy. But I contend that the proof of the pudding is in the eating. My patients give me conclusive and steadfast evidence that what I say about obesity control is clinically correct.

It is surprising to note the number of people who lose all their aches and pains and stiffness of the knees once their digestive combustion has improved. Those who have non-functioning gall bladders, and even people with gallstones, need have no misgivings about the diet I have been describing. So long as they take the medicines which these conditions call for, they can eat as I recommend. I have treated people with these afflictions, and if they stay on my diet, they feel better.

If you are seriously embarking on an obesity control regimen, a thorough medical check is highly recommended. For one thing, it would be well to determine just what weight it is desirable for you to be brought down to. Besides obvious considerations of height and age, there may be other factors that should be brought into focus such as the amount of recreation you get, your occupation, and whether you are a worrisome type, or are emotionally rugged. A physician can also advise if medication is desirable. In a few cases, a prescription relating to the glands' functioning will be in order. Prescriptions for other purposes may also be advisable in certain cases. Under no circumstances should you prescribe medicine for yourself or permit some well-meaning, misguided friend to talk you into taking some nostrum or patent medicine.

Your doctor, of course, can also do a little motivating. This doesn't necessarily mean a full excursion into psychology. I, for example, try to make each of my patients feel that he is on the threshold of a new, healthier, and more rewarding life.

Give the doctor who is providing guidance your complete confidence. When obstacles to the program arise, you must let him decide how they shall be dealt with.

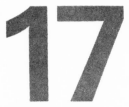

What You Can Look Forward to

EVERY INDIVIDUAL who follows the diet prescribed by me should ask himself the following questions:

> *Is my hunger satisfied?*
>
> *Am I sleeping well?*
>
> *Are my bowels and kidneys functioning as they should?*
>
> *Do I tire when I exercise?*

My diet is intended to rebuild the body. Of course, you will lose weight. Your clothes will become loose. You'll feel as light and springy as a gazelle.

Your weight should come down at the rate of two or three pounds a week. Your suit or dress size should change rapidly. How rapidly is indicated by examples taken, at random, from my case records.

>*Report A:* Dress 20½ in April; 18½ in July; 15 in October, 13 in February.

>*Report B:* Size 16 in January; 12 in June.

>*Report C:* A 44 waist in October; 40 in July.

>*Report D:* A 48 waist in May; 40 the next April.

Wardrobe replacement is one of the salient consequences of the no-starch diet. Yet, in all my time, I never heard a patient complain that this was a nuisance and an expense. They love it!

However, while the results of improving the body's thermostat adjustment are so apparent in the fit of clothing, the results are not to be discerned in sunken cheeks, hollow eyes, folds of unfilled skin, and other evidences of a starvation diet. The patient who stands before a mirror will have nothing but memory, or perhaps an old photograph, to tell him where he carried the weight which has disappeared.

Moreover, it will not be through changed appearance alone that the person who has rid himself of obesity through the process I have described will find satisfaction. Other good things will start to happen to him long before he has attained his weight goal. Stairs will be climbed without puffing. Energy will be left for pleasurable pursuits. Smarter dress will become a possibility. Personal confidence will reach a new high. As one of my patients wrote, "With the improvement of my physical appearance, everything else seems to have improved with it."

Or as another said, "I have more energy than I have had in 15 years. My nerves are calm. For the first time in 10 years, life is worth living."

Such remarks as these—and my files are full of them—are not testimonials to a miracle cure. The satisfactions of which they tell come from consistent adherence to a medically-premised regulation of the human system for the control of a disease called obesity. For the conscientious—and among my patients they have been the big majority—the great day finally comes. Milady has gone from 236 pounds and a 24½ dress to 136 pounds and a size 12. Once more she finds herself whistled at. What a welcome compliment!

I have given you a blueprint. That's all I can do. From now on, you know what your basic diet must be. But memory can be short, and the food-addicted can stray. These promised satisfactions will need to be recalled again and again by the determined dieter. The temptations to go astray will come with predictable certainty. You may go off the reservation and regain a few pounds. If it's only two or three, don't be alarmed. This can be controlled by increased recreation, and a slight cutback in starches. *I cannot stress enough the point that obesity is a continuous condition you must live with for a life-time. Never, never quit your basic diet!*

Actually, keeping a permanent limit on starches is not likely to prove inconvenient to the patient. I have found that the average person whom I treat has lost his appetite for starches. Most sincere dieters acquire a mistrust of starchy food which prompts them to avoid these foods even without my insistence.

For perhaps a year after attaining a much more slender figure, the patient should go on seeing his doctor once every three months or so. Such periodic checkups have a useful psychological purpose. A patient is much less likely to grow careless and start regaining weight if he must display the result of his lapses to his physician.

Some 70 percent of my patients succeed on their diet and *stay* successful. I have yet to hear of another weight-reduction regimen that can come near that mark—especially on the score of permanent poundage loss.

What can you look forward to if you slim down in the prescribed manner? Let me quote a letter from one of my former patients:

> *"I enjoy perfect health. I sleep well. Tiredness never affects me, whereas formerly after a little job of housework I had to lie down and rest. Formerly, just walking up our basement steps I would be out of breath and my heart would pound. I have not been nervous during the entire time. I can work and walk all day and be fresh to enter into evening activities with friends."*

Another wrote the following:

> "I am very happy with the results. I
> can wear a size 12 dress (was 20) or suit,
> and some size 10 dresses. Weight was
> 183, now 136. I am in good health. My
> blood pressure and heart are good. I can
> run up and downstairs without panting.
> I feel 10 years younger, too. Another
> nice thing about this diet is that you
> don't wrinkle even though you are not a
> girl anymore. I'm 48.
>
> "My waist has gone from 40½ to
> 36½. My biggest bad habit is eating
> between meals when I am home with
> nothing to do. I repeatedly tell my
> friends I have never felt so good in many
> years."

And still another enthusiast sent in the following letter:

> "I feel 100 percent stronger. Prior to
> this I could stand no exertion without
> feeling weak and dizzy. I also had to
> take cortisone daily for years for arthri-
> tis in my knees. Since using this plan, I
> have discontinued using cortisone alto-
> gether. I never feel weak or dizzy or
> have headaches. My blood pressure has
> dropped from 210 to 136."

The above are typical of the hundreds of letters that I have received from grateful patients who have found a new life. You will, too.

Index